DON'T TELL HER TO
RELAX

22 WAYS TO SUPPORT
YOUR INFERTILE LOVED ONE
THROUGH DIAGNOSIS, TREATMENT, AND BEYOND

ZAHIE EL KOURI

ISBN: 978-1-63192-805-5

TABLE OF CONTENTS

PROLOGUE

If you are reading this book, you have a loved one you either know or suspect is infertile.

In fact, 12 percent of all women of childbearing age struggle with infertility, or one in eight couples. This percentage is even higher for older women. About one-third of women over thirty-five have trouble getting pregnant.

But despite the fact that so many women struggle to have a child, most of them feel alone, in part because those closest to them don't know what to say or how to say it. Perhaps you are one of these people. You don't want to offend your friend; you don't want to make her sad; you don't want to intrude on her privacy. But you also don't want her to feel alone. You want to offer love and support and the opportunity to discuss what she is going through.

I've been on both sides of this predicament. I went through several years of fertility treatments and miscarriages before giving birth to my first child in 2011. I saw my friends and family struggle to know what to say and how to support me. I have also watched myself try and often fail to be as supportive as I would like of my friends who have struggled with infertility. To be specific, almost everything I suggest you *not* say to your infertile loved one, I myself have said and then regretted.

Does she want you to ignore her condition, or should you start a conversation about it? How does she want you to handle Mother's Day? Should you share your concerns about fertility treatments? What if fertility treatments don't work and she decides to adopt or live child-free instead?

This book will act as an intermediary between you and your Infertile Loved One (or ILO, for short), helping you walk the line between supportive and intrusive during her experience of infertility diagnosis, treatment, and beyond. It will tell you both what to say and do, and what *not* to say and do, while your Infertile Loved One is struggling to build her family.

Note to readers:

This book is written primarily for those who have a female loved one who is suffering from infertility. This is not to minimize the experience of male infertility, which is a very real problem with its own set of emotional, physical, and logistical challenges that deserves its own book.

In addition, the current edition of this book does not directly explore the issues particular to same-sex couples who are experiencing infertility and/ or using assisted reproductive technologies, although I do believe that much of the advice included here could be useful to those with GLBT loved ones in these situations.

More needs to be written about supporting both of these populations in their quests to have children. If you have recommendations you would like included in a future edition of this book, please contact me through my website, www.zahieelkouri.com.

CHAPTER 1

Understand What Infertility Really Means

The first thing you can do to help your loved one is to understand at least a little about the definition of infertility. According to the American Society for Reproductive Medicine, infertility is "a disease defined by the failure to achieve a successful pregnancy after twelve months or more of regular unprotected intercourse."

For women over age thirty-five, the numbers change, and infertility is defined by the failure to achieve a successful pregnancy after six months. If your loved one has been trying to get pregnant for only a few months, she is not yet infertile. If she meets the six- or twelve-month cutoff, then she has become your Infertile Loved One (ILO), and some or all of the following tips may help you support her in the days and months to come.

Infertility can have a variety of medical causes, including endometriosis, luteal phase defect, male factor challenges, ovulatory disorders, polycystic ovarian syndrome, premature ovarian failure, uterine abnormalities, or chromosomal abnormalities of the embryos themselves. (See the end of this chapter for descriptions of these causes.) Your ILO might find a diagnosis of a medical cause reassuring, but she might also feel angry and disappointed that she can't get pregnant like everyone else.

From time to time, your ILO may forget that infertility is a medical problem and try to blame herself. She might do this despite any of the previous diagnoses, or because of the dreaded and frustrating diagnosis of

Unexplained Infertility. One in five couples get this lack of a diagnosis. If she is over thirty-five and trying to get pregnant, her doctor may identify her as a woman of Advanced Reproductive Age and explain to her that her chances of conceiving are much lower than if she were in her twenties, specifically because chromosomal abnormalities are simply more likely in embryos formed from older eggs.

Your loved one may talk about her difficulty conceiving as being her fault. You may hear her say this after a failed fertility treatment, after a miscarriage, or even after diagnosis. Other friends might tell her she has simply waited too long to try to get pregnant. If she goes through a fertility workup, the doctor may not find a cause of her infertility. All this can make her feel terrible and guilty and scared that she will not be able to get pregnant and have a child.

Remind her of all the medical advice she has followed and all the dedication she has shown in her quest to become a parent. You can also gently remind her that most failed fertility treatments and early miscarriages are the result of chromosomal abnormalities, which are, of course, not her fault. If she is over thirty-five, and says that she waited too long to try to get pregnant, help her focus on the future rather than the past. If it is appropriate, remind her that she was looking for the right partner with whom to have a child.

••

Takeaway Tip: Use the information in this book to help your ILO remember that infertility usually has a medical cause and is not her fault.

••

COMMON MEDICAL CAUSES OF INFERTILITY

Endometriosis is a disorder of the female reproductive system in which endometrial tissue (the normal lining of the uterus) is found outside the uterine cavity. An estimated three to five million American women of reproductive age suffer from endometriosis. This disease is most common in women 30-40 years of age, though it can begin in the late teens and early twenties. About 40 percent of patients with endometriosis will experience some degree of infertility.

Luteal phase defect means that the lining of the uterus is not getting adequately prepared to support an embryo at the appropriate time in the menstrual cycle.

Ovulatory disorders exist when hormonal imbalances cause problems with the thyroid or the pituitary, leading to changes in timing or sufficiency of ovulation.

Polycystic ovarian syndrome is both one of the most underdiagnosed medical conditions in the United States and one of the leading causes of infertility. It is often very treatable by controlling the patient's insulin levels and using medication to trigger ovulation.

Premature ovarian failure is the cessation of menstrual periods before the age of forty. While there are relatively few treatment options that restore ovulation, patients can sometimes get pregnant with donor eggs or donor embryos.

Uterine abnormalities are structural problems of the uterus, whether from a congenital defect or as the result of surgery or infection; they can often be corrected with surgery.

Male factor infertility: 35 percent of infertility is related to male factor problems such as structural abnormalities, sperm production disorders, ejaculatory disturbances and immunologic disorders.

Chromosomal abnormalities of the embryos themselves can cause a woman to have trouble getting and/or staying pregnant. By this I mean that sperm and egg are coming together to create an embryo, but that embryo doesn't develop normally. Chromosomal abnormalities in embryos become more common as women get older, but even young women can experience infertility and miscarriage for this reason. If the chromosomes of an embryo are abnormal, there is really nothing your ILO or her doctor can do to save the pregnancy and ensure the birth of a healthy baby. In fact, over half of all pregnancies end because of chromosomal abnormalities very early, sometimes even before the woman knows she is pregnant. Knowing this may reassure your ILO that her failure to get or stay pregnant is not because of something she is or is not doing.

CHAPTER 2

Keep an Open Mind
about Babies

If you suspect that your loved one is having trouble getting pregnant, you may want to offer your support right away, but the most supportive thing you can do is wait for her to bring the subject up.

Your loved one may have made the decision to live a full life without children and may be troubled by the reminder that you might expect otherwise. If your loved one wants children and hasn't mentioned them, she might have decided that now is just not the right time. And if your loved one is trying to get pregnant and has not succeeded, she may not be ready to discuss the subject at this time.

Sometimes, well-meaning friends and relatives want their loved ones to experience the same joy in parenthood that they did. They might ask, "When are you going to have a baby?" If they know, either anecdotally or through research, that a woman's fertility decreases with age, they might even say, "You're not getting any younger!"

If you are one of these friends or relatives, you might mean no harm, but your ILO will likely find these statements hurtful. The truth is that we live in an information age. Your loved one probably knows that fertility decreases with age. If she has a husband or partner, or has made the decision to have a child on her own, she has probably already contemplated the timing of getting pregnant. She may not feel ready to share this very personal information with anyone.

So how can you reach out without offending her?

If you know your loved one is trying to get pregnant but isn't talking about it, consider saying: "I know you are hoping to start a family. If you ever need any advice or support, I am here for you in whatever way you need."

If you absolutely cannot hold your tongue—if your curiosity is causing you physical pain, and you MUST know whether your loved one wants a baby—ask, "Are you interested in having children?" rather than "When are you having a baby?"

If your loved one says no, then you have your answer. If your loved one says "We'll see," or "Someday," you can say, "If you ever need advice or support, I am here for you." Trust your ILO to make good decisions and to ask for your advice and support when she needs it.

• •

Takeaway Tip: Never ask, "When are you going to have a baby?" Instead ask, "Are you interested in having children?" Otherwise, say nothing at all.

• •

CHAPTER 3

Empathize with Your Infertile Loved One's Sense of Urgency

While many women won't want to discuss their infertility, some will eventually confide in close friends or relatives, and others will be open about their difficulties with getting pregnant from the first sign of trouble.

If you know your ILO is having trouble getting pregnant, whether she has told you or you just suspect, it may be very tempting to tell her to relax. You are not alone. As a society we seem to have decided that, "Just relax and you'll get pregnant," should be the automatic response to a confession of infertility.

Variations on the theme include, "If you go on a vacation, I just know you will get pregnant."

Or, "If you start the adoption process, you will get pregnant."

Or, "The minute you stop trying to get pregnant, you will get pregnant for sure." All of these statements sound fine in the abstract.

It's true that many women get pregnant while waiting to be placed with a child through adoption. It's true that relaxation is key to good health, and good health is important for the reproductive system. It's true that vacations are generally excellent, and your ILO probably deserves one.

But the reality is that true infertility is a medical condition, and relaxation will not cure any of the underlying physiological problems that cause it. Adoption is a long process, and some women will get pregnant while waiting to be placed with a child just because of how long it takes.

But if your ILO has primary ovarian insufficiency (formerly known as premature ovarian failure), no amount of relaxation or adoption paperwork will help her conceive a child.

Even if your ILO knows you mean well, try to hold off from offering this kind of advice. It can sound flippant and smug, even if you don't mean it that way. And even if relaxation would help, your directive will not help your ILO relax at all, and will probably make her feel as though you don't understand her sense of urgency and panic about having a child, in turn making her feel less supported rather than more supported in her situation.

• •

Takeaway Tip: Never say, "Just relax, and you'll get pregnant." Concentrate on other aspects of your relationship, or gently ask, "Do you want to talk about your fertility treatments?" You can always remind your ILO of the following: "I want you to know that I am not bringing up babies because I don't want to be nosy, but if you ever want to talk about them, I'm here for you."

• •

CHAPTER 4

Send Fertile Thoughts Rather than
Making Promises about Motherhood

If you suspect that your ILO is having difficulty conceiving a child, avoid saying, "I just know you will be a mother soon." Avoid any promise of motherhood.

You mean well. Probably you can't imagine that this person you love will *not* become a mother. But you might inadvertently be upsetting your ILO.

This kind of promise, no matter how well intended, is not what she needs to hear.

Remember, there are no guarantees with fertility treatments. Your ILO may never get pregnant with her own eggs. She may never get pregnant, and may choose to adopt. Then again, she may try to adopt, but never be able to finalize an adoption.

Here are some specific times when you might be especially tempted to make this kind of promise or prediction:

On Mother's Day: You may be at a loss for what to say to your ILO. You know she wants a child, and you suspect that Mother's Day might be difficult for her. You might be tempted to say, "By this time next year, you will be a mother."

Consider instead saying just what you are thinking: "I know today must be difficult for you. If you want to talk about it, I am here for you."

In the middle of a medicated fertility cycle: Once you've watched your ILO give herself a thousand shots to hyper-stimulate her ovaries for an in vitro fertilization (IVF) cycle, and listened to her story of a successful egg retrieval, it might seem inevitable to you that all this effort will result in a child.

But not all IVF cycles work. In fact, depending on several factors, there's actually less than a 50 percent chance that the first cycle will give your ILO a baby. So it is probably safer to say, "I'm sending fertile thoughts your way," than to say, "I just know this cycle will work for you and you will get pregnant."

Unfortunately, many IVF cycles will not work. Some couples will go through several IVF cycles or donor egg cycles before they conceive a child, while other couples will never conceive a child at all.

••

Takeaway Tip: Even though it's often tricky, try to be supportive without guaranteeing success. Don't say, "I just know you'll be a mother soon." Say, "I'm sending fertile thoughts your way." Or, if you are religious, "I'm praying for you."

••

The Society for Assisted Reproductive Technology reports that the success rates for a single cycle of non-donor egg IVF nationwide are as follows:

- 42.5% in women younger than 35 years of age
- 34.5% in women aged 35-37 years
- 24.2% in women aged 38-40 years
- 13.3% in women aged 41-42 years
- 5.6% in women aged 43-44 years

*These are the 2013 number for retrievals using fresh embryos rather than frozen embryos and resulting in live birth. For more detailed information, please visit the SART website.

CHAPTER 5

Adopt a Careful Tone When Talking about Adoption

Adoption is a great blessing for many families, whether or not they have gone through infertility. You probably know someone who has adopted or has been adopted, and you want your ILO to know how great adoption can turn out. You may wonder why your ILO is putting herself through this physical and hormonal boot camp when there are so many children in the world who need parents.

This is why so many people ask, "Why don't you just adopt?" when they find out someone is having trouble getting pregnant or is going through fertility treatments.

Remember, we live in an information age, so your ILO knows that adoption is an option. She may already have considered it. She may have looked at the IVF protocols and been daunted by the sheer number of needles involved, and come to the conclusion that she would rather adopt. She may have already researched both domestic and international adoption, and gone to meet with an adoption agency or even had a home study. In the course of this research, she may have discovered that she or her partner don't qualify to adopt, which can be true because of age or health or other reasons. She may have become nervous about a birth mother changing her mind later in the process. She may have already gone through an adoption attempt, and ended up with heartbreak and no baby. Or perhaps she and her partner discussed adoption early on and decided that having a child who shared their genetics was important to them. They may not have ruled out adoption, but they want to try IVF first. In that case, your ILO may feel like anyone who brings up adoption is second-guessing her choices, rather than supporting her in her current path.

If you know that your ILO is struggling with infertility and is either considering or going through fertility treatments, hold off on discussing adoption. At some point, after you and your ILO have discussed her desire for parenthood at length, you might be able to broach the subject. But first, consider your motivation. Are you genuinely trying to help your ILO find the best path to parenthood for her situation, or are you thinking more about what you might choose to do in the same situation?

••

Takeaway Tip: Instead of asking, "Why don't you just adopt?" ask, "Is adoption something you might be interested in?" If you feel like you may have strong feelings about adoption, one way or another, that would inhibit your ability to be sensitive and supportive about the issue, consider not bringing it up at all.

••

CHAPTER 6

Understand the Emotional, Logistical, and Financial Challenges of Fertility Treatments

By now, you have probably heard of someone getting pregnant through in vitro fertilization, or IVF. If you know your loved one is having trouble getting pregnant, it may seem obvious to you that she should move on to IVF. It is true that for many women, and many couples, IVF can significantly increase the chances of getting pregnant.

> **In vitro fertilization (IVF)** is a process in which a woman gives herself injections to hyper-stimulate her ovaries for the development of multiple eggs. A doctor then harvests, or removes, those eggs and fertilizes them in a petri dish with sperm from the woman's partner or a sperm donor. Three or five days later, the doctor puts the developing embryos back inside the woman's uterus, where they continue to grow.

First, let's talk about the reason you shouldn't bring IVF up in this particular way: No one wants to hear that they need medical help getting pregnant. Most women would prefer to get pregnant in an intimate setting with their partner, by candlelight and romantic music, rather than with the assistance of daily hormone shots, a speculum, a laboratory, and several dozen healthcare professionals. So even if IVF is exactly what she needs, you can help your ILO by leaving it to her doctor to bring up IVF when and if it becomes appropriate.

Next, let's talk about why IVF might not be the best path for your ILO. IVF is an invasive, expensive process, and for most women, there are actually other treatments worth trying first. Some women will be able to get pregnant using fertility treatments that stop short of IVF, which might include oral medications, injectable medications, minimally invasive office procedures, and even surgery. Other women will decide they don't want any medical intervention at all, whether for religious or other reasons.

What does this mean for you? The best way you can support your ILO is to encourage her to get the best medical evaluation possible, which usually means seeing a specialist. If your ILO tells you she is considering seeing a doctor to talk about her difficulty getting pregnant, rather than asking about IVF right away, you can help her by asking whether she has made an appointment with a board-certified reproductive endocrinologist.

According to The Society of Reproductive Endocrinology & Infertility (SREI), a subdivision of the American Society for Reproductive Medicine, your ILO should seek the care of a reproductive endocrinologist if she is under the age of thirty-five and unable to achieve pregnancy after twelve months of unprotected intercourse, or if she is thirty-five or older and has been trying for more than six months. Your ILO may get all the care she needs from her gynecologist, but a board-certified reproductive endocrinologist is better equipped to evaluate her, run the appropriate tests on both her and her partner, and advise her on all her options.

If your ILO does turn to IVF, she is crossing a line from what might have been a private and romantic path to parenthood to a less personal, more technological path, with all the physical, financial, and emotional challenges that medical fertility treatment entails. Be aware that she may need to mourn her imagined path to conception, and she may want to do so in private.

• •

Takeaway Tip: Instead of saying, "Why don't you just do IVF?" say, "Do you think you would consider fertility treatments?" or "Have you thought about meeting with a specialist to explore all your options?"

• •

CHAPTER 7

Be a Secret Agent

If your ILO has confided in you about her difficulty getting pregnant, you may be one of a select few. Some women are very open about fertility challenges and treatments, but many choose to only discuss them with a few trusted friends. By being in the know, you can help your ILO in a variety of ways, kind of like a covert operative or secret agent.

To begin with, if you know that your ILO is sensitive to other women's fertility, you can cover for her at baby showers or any other gathering where everyone is talking about babies or might ask her when she is planning to get pregnant, either by helping her brainstorm a polite excuse not to attend, or by coming along, standing at her side during the gathering, and changing the subject politely whenever anyone gets too close to a difficult topic. If your ILO is able to decline the invitation, offer to take her out to lunch or to a movie to help keep her mind off any grief or disappointment she might be experiencing.

If you are hosting these gatherings, don't leave your ILO out—make sure to invite her to every family birthday party and Mother's Day celebration, and to send her an invitation to your baby shower—but also make a special call or send a special e-mail telling her she is welcome but you will understand if she doesn't want to attend. If you are technologically savvy, offer to text photos and videos during the event so that she doesn't miss anything but is not subjected to happy pregnant women or well-meaning Aunt Martha, who will keep asking why she doesn't have a baby.

Another way you can help your ILO is by conducting surveillance on fertile friends. I'm not suggesting you actually wiretap anyone, but you can pay extra attention to telltale signs of pregnancy, like whether your mutual friends are avoiding sushi and soft cheeses. If you find out that a mutual friend or family member is pregnant, the best thing you can do for your ILO is to let her know in private. She may not be bothered by such news, but it may make her more upset than she can predict. By giving her advance notice, you can let her figure out her emotions without a large public audience.

You can also use your special position as confidant to help your ILO gather information about healthcare professionals. Your ILO might love to find a local reproductive endocrinologist, or the right support group, but she might not want to make her infertility public by asking her other friends or acquaintances for recommendations. You can help by acting as an intermediary. You can ask friends if they have heard anything about local (and national) reproductive endocrinologists and fertility clinics without using your ILO's name.

Sometimes your ILO will need the company of friends and family, but sometimes she won't want to speak to anyone who is not also going through fertility treatments. Family gatherings and baby showers may be especially stressful. The emotional, physical, financial, and social pressures of infertility often feel overwhelming. Your ILO may no longer have the emotional bandwidth she once had to deal with other people. She may need some time alone to regroup, possibly on the bathroom floor. If you are a texting sort of person, send her supportive texts or e-mails that say something like, "Here for you. Talk babies or politics or latest starlet gossip?"

If your ILO has taken her phone or computer into the bathroom with her, she might burst into tears, but she will appreciate your support.

If she has left her technology behind, she will find your messages when she emerges from her cocoon, and she will know she has your support for whatever comes next.

••

Takeaway Tip: Use your special position as confidant to help your ILO navigate challenging social situations.

••

CHAPTER 8:

Educate Yourself about the Infertility Workup

If you know your ILO is visiting a reproductive endocrinologist, you can support her by educating yourself about the kinds of appointments and tests that may be in her future.

Your ILO may not want to discuss these with you, but if she does, you will be better prepared for it. If she doesn't, you will have a better sense of how intense and overwhelming these appointments can be.

At your ILO's first appointment, her doctor will take a thorough medical history, asking lots of questions about menstruation, past sexual partners, birth control, current sexual practices, and other surgical and medical treatments.

The doctor will also likely do a physical exam at this visit, including a thyroid exam and a transvaginal ultrasound. Even if your ILO was excited about getting help with conceiving, she may be surprised and upset by how much privacy she must surrender in just this first appointment.

Either during this first appointment or on day three of her next menstrual cycle, your ILO will go in to her doctor's office or another facility for a blood draw, which may be the first of many. At some point, your ILO may need to have one or more of the following:

- Hysterosalpingogram (HSG): An HSG is an x-ray procedure per-formed in the first half of the cycle, using water- or oil-based dye to identify any structural abnormalities in the uterus or fallopian tubes. This procedure is sometimes done in a doctor's office, but may also be done in a hospital by a radiologist. This could mean that your ILO will be wide awake with her legs spread apart in a procedure room while a doctor puts a speculum in her vagina and injects liquid into her uterus. This procedure may cause mild cramping, so it can be uncomfortable, and even if your ILO does not feel the cramping, it may interfere with the ability to deter-mine what is going on and make the test longer.

- Sonohystogram (also known as a Sonohysterogram): A doctor fills the uterine cavity with saline before an ultrasound for careful examination of the uterus.

- Hysteroscopy: A doctor examines the uterus for abnormali-ties using a tiny telescope mounted with a fiber optic light. For many people, this is a painless procedure, so most doctors do not prescribe any sort of anesthesia or sedation, but this means that if your ILO is in the minority of women who find it extremely pain-ful, she may be traumatized.

- Laparoscopy: While your ILO is under anesthesia, her doctor makes a few small incisions in her abdomen and uses a laparo-scope to examine the ovaries, fallopian tubes, and uterus. If the doctor finds endometriosis or adhesions, she may remove them with a special laser.

· ·

Takeaway Tip: *Learning about a typical fertility workup*
will help you better empathize with your ILO and support her.

· ·

CHAPTER 9

Offer Company and Transportation

A fertility workup can take up a lot of time, with many different trips to the doctor's office, and sometimes even the hospital, for different tests.

If your ILO ends up moving on to other fertility treatments, she will have even more appointments to attend, including early-morning blood draws and frequent examinations.

If your ILO tells you she is having any of these procedures, you can support her by offering to drive her to and from her appointment or by meeting her at the medical office prior to the appointment. If your ILO is having a laparoscopy, she will be under general anesthesia, and will definitely need a ride to and from the hospital or clinic.

This gesture can provide valuable support whether or not your ILO has a partner. Sometimes there are just so many appointments to attend that her partner might need a break to take care of other matters. (Note that since some of these visits are invasive, your ILO might prefer that you stay in the waiting room while she goes in for procedures alone, but might still appreciate the company to and from the appointment.)

If you cannot join her for her appointments, consider buying her a trashy magazine to entertain her while she's waiting.

If your ILO gets further along in fertility treatments and needs surgery, or has an intrauterine insemination or in vitro fertilization, she might need bed rest or modified bed rest (or general stay-at- home-on-your- couch rest). You can support your ILO by asking if she'd like you to bring over dinner or a movie, or whether you can come over for a cup of tea and a visit. And if this bed or couch rest is your ILO's idea and not her doctor's, you can support her by not second-guessing her decision to limit her activities.

••

Takeaway Tip: Remember, your company is usually worth more to your ILO than any specific comment or piece of advice. Offer to help out however she needs and be prepared to just listen and be supportive.

••

CHAPTER 10:

Be Aware of the Effects of Fertility Hormones

Most fertility patients will take some form of hormones during their treatment. Some women will be able to start by taking pills like clomiphene or letrozole, and others will take a mix of pills and injections. Often the cycle will start with one month of birth control pills.

Your ILO may take these hormones as part of a cycle during which her doctor advises her to have sex at a particular time, or as part of an intrauterine insemination. She will definitely use injectable hormones for an IVF cycle.

For each different path and patient, doctors will prescribe different dosages and combinations of hormones, depending on the situation and how sensitive the patient is to the drug.

Taking fertility drugs is a roller coaster. If you are a woman who has ever menstruated, imagine your worst menstrual cycle ever, and multiply your physical and emotional symptoms by one thousand. If you have never been subject to the hormones of a menstrual cycle, then imagine your worst day ever, and your best day ever, and imagine them in a repeat cycle every four minutes.

Your ILO may be perfectly composed during the whole cycle, or she may turn into a fire-breathing bitch, or she may get extra cuddly and amorous, or she may burst into tears at the first frame of a cotton commercial.

It is very possible that she may exhibit each of these behaviors in twenty-minute increments for the entire duration of her fertility treatments.

None of these behaviors is her fault. Keep reminding yourself of this, even as she's weeping over a carton of eggs at the grocery store. Offer white chocolate (so as to help her avoid caffeine). Take her to a funny movie. Rather than saying, "You are just hormonal," say, "I'm desperate to see the new Channing Tatum movie—can you please keep me company?" Then show up at the theater with a feather boa.

••

Takeaway Tip: Your ILO will probably be cranky and emotional during fertility treatments because of the medicines she is taking. Remember that the medicines are causing her physical and emotional challenges and she may not be herself again until she stops taking them. Ask if there is anything you can do to help, and be patient with any emotional volatility.

••

CHAPTER 11

Educate Yourself about Invasive Treatments Like IUI and IVF

One minute you and your ILO speak the same language, and the next she is talking in acronyms: FSH (Follicle Stimulating Hormone), PCOS (Polycystic Ovarian Syndrome), BFN (Big Fat Negative, as in the big fat negative or minus sign one sees on a home pregnancy test); BFP (the Big Fat Positive sign your ILO is hoping for), IUI, and IVF. These last two are particular medical procedures that can help your ILO get pregnant. By learning about IUIs and IVFs, you can better support your ILO.

An **IUI** is an intrauterine insemination, a process in which a doctor places sperm in your ILO's uterus while she is ovulating. It is like a protracted pelvic exam. Several hours before the actual insemination, your ILO's husband or male partner (or donor) will supply the sperm so it can be spun through a centrifuge and concentrated into a vial of super-sperm; only the best and brightest are given that special head start past the cervix. Sometimes this can be done without any medications, but often there will at least be a shot to trigger ovulation, and sometimes other shots to increase the number of eggs released during the cycle. (Remember that only one egg is usually released per cycle. In a medicated IUI, the goal might be to stimulate the growth of two or three eggs.)

After an insemination, your ILO will usually rest for twenty or thirty minutes and then spend the next two weeks waiting for the results of a pregnancy test. (This period is called the Two-Week Wait, which is important to know because your ILO might start sending you e-mails talking about "the TWW" as though you, too, speak in the language of infertility acronyms.)

An **IVF** (in vitro fertilization) cycle combines the emotional roller coaster of fertility shots with the intrusion of the IUI and adds in conscious sedation and an egg retrieval. In a medicated IUI, the goal is to stimulate the growth of only two or three eggs, but in most IVF cycles the goal is to produce many more so you have enough for several attempts at pregnancy.

An IVF cycle might begin with a month of birth control pills or other medication, and then seven to twelve days of medicines to stimulate extra ovulation. When your ILO's ovarian follicles get to a certain size, and just before they are released through ovulation, her reproductive endocrinologist will "retrieve" all the eggs of a promising size. This is surgery, and your ILO will be under conscious sedation. She may be sore afterwards and will probably receive a prescription for pain medication. The eggs retrieved will then be introduced to the sperm sample and watched closely for the next few days. The IVF lab will report back to your ILO periodically and let her know how many of the eggs have been fertilized, and then how many of those embryos are growing properly.

Just a few short years ago, the usual practice was for your ILO to go back to the clinic or hospital and have an intrauterine transfer, this time of one or more embryos, but now it is more typical for all the embryos to be vitrified, or frozen, and for your ILO to return for transfer in a later cycle.

Distract your ILO during the Implantation Window.

After both an insemination and an embryo transfer, your ILO may go about her business as usual, but she may want to take it easy for a few days. Many doctors say you don't need to limit your activity, and that you can even exercise as usual, but some recommend bed rest for forty-eight hours. Some fertility patients will find comfort in the idea that there is nothing they can do to disrupt the fertilization and implantation, and others will want to be as cautious as possible and stay in bed for the weekend. You can support your ILO by keeping her company during this time.

Distract your ILO during the Two-Week Wait. No matter whether your ILO had an IUI or a frozen transfer of IVF embryos, she may have complicated emotions around the two-week wait between the procedure and her pregnancy test. In a frozen embryo transfer, depending on the number of days the embryos are allowed to grow in vitro, there will be about nine to fourteen days between transfer and the first pregnancy test. After either procedure, your ILO will have to observe all the protocols of pregnancy without knowing whether she is pregnant.

Women deal with the Two-Week Wait in different ways. Some will be unrelentingly optimistic, while others will feel depressed and hopeless, as if thinking the worst will help protect them from possible bad news.

Why does you knowing the difference between IUI and IVF help your ILO?

These two procedures may not seem very different to you, but they may seem hugely different to your ILO. For one thing, IUIs might be covered by insurance, while IVF is only covered by insurance in a handful of states. In addition, many people have ethical or religious concerns about creating embryos in a lab. Starting IUIs may have been emotionally difficult, but moving on to IVF may seem like an enormous step. And whether or not your ILO is having trouble with the decision, she will be comforted if you use the correct terms for the procedures she has chosen.

....

Takeaway Tip: Knowing the difference between IUI and IVF cycles will help you know what your ILO is going through during particular steps in the process.

....

CHAPTER 12

Help with Shots

If your ILO is having a medicated IUI or is moving on to IVF, she or a loved one will have to give her a number of shots. She will have to do this on a particular schedule, usually twice a day. These shots are usually administered in the abdomen or posterior. Many of them require special mixing or preparation, which might cause your ILO to feel overwhelmed or like an amateur chemist.

There are four different ways you can help your ILO at this stage: research, giving the shots, preparing the shots, and offering your company.

Research. If research is your thing, you might help your ILO by asking her the names of all the drugs she will need to inject and finding online videos of women preparing and giving themselves the shots. You can put all the links or files in one convenient e-mail so she does not have to look for them if she needs instruction or reassurance during her daily ritual. Most fertility clinics offer a training session for each fertility patient, but it can still be unnerving to give yourself the shots on your own.

Play doctor (or more accurately, nurse). If you are a healthcare professional or are especially brave, and your ILO mentions that she wishes someone else would give her the shots, you can help her by offering to play doctor. There are some shots that a fertility patient can give herself, but others, like the progesterone-in-oil shots many women need for several days after an embryo transfer, are almost impossible to give oneself because of their location on the backside. Many husbands and partners give their ILO fertility injections with minimal training, so you are likely just as qualified as anyone else. If both your ILO and her husband or partner are afraid of needles, they might be especially grateful to have a close friend or relative help them with this challenge. If your ILO does take you up on your offer, know that the actual moment of the shot may not bother some women, but others will find some relief in icing the area before the injection. If you offer and your ILO respectfully declines, that's okay too.

Play chemist. For some ILOs, the act of giving the shot is not difficult, but the mixing of the powders with liquid and the drawing up of the syringe feels like too much high school chemistry. Your ILO may appreciate your offer to read all the instructions, watch the videos, and give her a day or two off from being responsible for preparing all the injectable medications she needs to take.

Admire your ILO's medical skills. If research, chemistry, and medical procedures are not up your alley, consider offering your ILO your company during this process of preparing and giving herself injections. In particular, she might appreciate the fact that someone she is close to really understands all that she is doing in her efforts to have a child.

You know your ILO best. If she is a more private person, she might prefer that you give her space while she gives herself the shots.

• •

Takeaway Tip: If your ILO tells you she is overwhelmed by some aspect of the shots required for IVF or sometimes for IUI, offer to help.

• •

CHAPTER 13

Offer to Be Chief Financial Officer of Your Infertile Loved One's Family Building Endeavor

IVF is expensive, and most states don't require insurance to cover it, so your ILO may be worried about funding her IVF cycles. The truth is IVF will probably never cost less than $10,000. If your ILO confides that she is worried about the cost of IVF, there are a few ways you can help.

Research. You can offer to research IVF funding. Resolve: The National Infertility Association has a fantastic website, crucial for many kinds of information. They have compiled comprehensive information about scholarships, financing programs, medical treatment package plans, and pro bono treatments at http://www.resolve.org/family-building-options/making-treatment-affordable.html. If your ILO agrees, you can comb through this information on her behalf, and even do some additional research about clinical trials.

Invest in your ILO's future parenthood. If you are related to your ILO, you might be happy to contribute money towards treatments. You might say, "I know IVF is very expensive. I have $2,000 set aside for a special occasion. I would love to offer it to you to help, no strings attached." Or you might offer her a no- or low-interest loan.

• •

Takeaway Tip: If you have time or money to contribute, consider helping your ILO out with the financial burden of fertility treatment.

• •

CHAPTER 14

Make a Care Package

If your ILO is undergoing treatments like IUI or IVF, or if she is having surgery, consider making her a care package. At any time during diagnosis or treatment, your ILO will appreciate a thoughtful gift.

You know your ILO, so you will know what kind of media she needs, whether that might be trashy magazines, a juicy paperback copy of *Anna Karenina*, or a gift card for iTunes.

If she is having an IUI or IVF, she will spend a lot of time with her feet in stirrups, naked from the waist down. One of the best ways you can support her is to buy her a cozy pair of socks—or, if you have knitting skills, consider making a pair from scratch. Socks are such a big deal with fertility treatments that one group of women organized a sock exchange to support each other during treatment (http://searchingforoursilverlining. blogspot.com/p/fertility-socks.html).

If you are more ambitious, and if your ILO is having IVF or a medicated IUI, you can make a medication box. For both IVF and medicated IUIs, your ILO has a lot of medication to keep track of. She will usually receive a large cardboard box in the mail, full of medicines, needles, syringes, and a sharps container for disposing of used needles. She will have to refrigerate some portion of these medicines, and store the rest of them. You can make her experience of injections more pleasant by decorating a box for her where she can store her needles, syringes, and drugs.

Better yet, make two—one for the needles and syringes and sharps container, and another for all the medications that need to be refrigerated.

••

Takeaway Tip: *Your ILO will appreciate any gesture or gift, especially if it shows you have found a little extra time to think about exactly what she is going through.*

••

CHAPTER 15

Understand the Ethics and Protocol of IVF Embryo Transfer

The celebrity of high-order multiples has really made life difficult for the infertile woman. The media coverage of women who give birth to six or eight babies after fertility treatments makes the general public believe that fertility treatments always involve such a risk. Often these risks are actually the first thing that comes to mind when one hears that a friend or loved one is considering any kind of fertility treatment. These well-meaning people are worried that having six or eight children in a single pregnancy is a real danger with conventional IVF treatment, and they know that the uterus simply cannot do a good job of gestating eight embryos at once. They don't want their ILO to go through what the women pregnant with those multiples went through, and they don't want their ILO's children to face the same health risks those higher-order multiples faced.

The truth is that the Society for Assisted Reproductive Technology (SART) has standards for how many embryos to transfer. An ethical doctor will only transfer more than two embryos if your ILO has already been through IVF and had poor results with getting pregnant, if she has had multiple miscarriages that the doctor suspects are the result of chromosomal abnormalities, or if she is of advanced reproductive age.

Even twin births are risky for most women, so the goal of most ethical doctors is a singleton birth. For this reason, in some other countries, you are only able to transfer one embryo at a time. In most states in the US insurance does not cover IVF, putting more financial pressure on the US

IVF patient to increase her chances of a live birth by transferring multiple embryos. Many women transfer two embryos at a time, and a few women choose to transfer more than two embryos at a time. To transfer more than two, the patient has to agree to selective reduction in case more than two or three embryos implant. An ethical doctor will give your ILO quite a long lecture about the risks of having multiples.

While you might think you are lightening the mood by mentioning celebrity multiples, your ILO may feel like you don't understand the dozens of hours she has spent thinking about how many embryos to transfer. She might welcome the chance to talk through the pros and cons of transferring more than one embryo, if you approach the subject in a serious, respectful, and genuinely curious way.

· ·

Takeaway Tip: Don't say, "Don't get pregnant with octuplets!"
Instead say, "I hear it is hard to decide how many embryos to transfer.
What number seems right to you?"

· ·

CHAPTER 16

Offer Childcare to Those Experiencing Secondary Infertility

According to the Center for Disease Control, about half of all infertility cases are secondary infertility, or cases in which a couple already has a child and has trouble conceiving a second child. Secondary infertility is just as emotionally complicated as primary infertility. Your ILO may have just as much attachment to the idea of giving her child a sibling as she had about having a child at all. She may not have had any difficulty conceiving a first child, but has suddenly found herself having difficulty conceiving a second child.

No matter your thoughts on whether being or having an only child is a good or bad thing, refrain from expressing your opinion unless your ILO asks you for it. Having a second child is just as much a personal decision as having a first child, and deserves just as much support. Saying, "At least you have one child," is never helpful to someone who wants a second child.

That said, your ILO may worry about spending so much time, money, and emotional energy on a hypothetical second child, and feel guilty about the effect of all of this on the first, existing child. You can help by offering to spend quality time with your ILO's first child and generally giving him or her a little extra attention.

• •

Takeaway Tip: Support your ILO though secondary infertility by offering to spend some time with her first child while she undergoes fertility testing or treatment to expand her family.

• •

CHAPTER 17

Respect Your Infertile Loved One's Dedication and Persistence

It may seem to you like everyone is getting pregnant through IVF. As more and more celebrities open up about assisted reproductive technology, IVF may seem like a sure thing. If your ILO does not get pregnant through IVF, you may think that a pregnancy is just not meant to be, or that her medical issues are not ones that IVF can circumvent. But many first IVF cycles fail, and they often provide valuable information to your ILO's doctors that will increase the likelihood of success with a second cycle.

If your ILO has only done one cycle of IVF, and it has failed, avoid suggesting that she should give up and move on. If your ILO goes through many cycles of fertility treatment, you may worry about her emotional and physical health and wonder if she should stop treatment. But it is only after a third failed cycle that chances of success start to decrease, and even then, this kind of analysis is best left to doctors, patients, and partners. If your ILO is ready to keep going, support her choice, even if it means having a more hormonal, less emotionally available friend for a while.

If you are the spouse or partner of the ILO, you might express that you are having a hard time with the cycle of hope and despair, and that you also need support in this process.

If your ILO does stop a particular kind of family-building measure, encourage her to not think of it as giving up. Rather, at every stage of the family-building process, encourage her to think about the positives of the next stage. If IVF doesn't work out and she turns to donor-egg, be excited about that prospect with her. If she decides to adopt, focus on the excitement of that process. And if she decides to stop pursuing parenthood, support her in that decision as well.

••

Takeaway Tip: Don't ask, "Isn't it time to give up?"
Instead ask, "What do you think you will do next?"

••

CHAPTER 18

Allow Your Infertile Loved One to Grieve

Allow your ILO to grieve a miscarriage or unsuccessful cycle or the loss of a twin during pregnancy. Fertility treatments do not equal pregnancy, and pregnancy does not equal the live birth of a baby. Many women will go through IVF and not get pregnant. Some women will get pregnant, but after a few days their hormone levels will go down and their doctor will tell them they had a "chemical pregnancy." Since this happens so early, it is the kind of pregnancy that your ILO would not even know she was experiencing if not for modern fertility treatments and blood test monitoring.

It is common for women to miscarry in the first few months of pregnancy, usually because of chromosomal abnormalities, but sometimes because of other problems. Miscarriage is difficult for most women, but for fertility patients, it can be even more difficult because of the brief glimmer of hope that pregnancy gave them.

An even more specific kind of grief comes when a fertility patient gets pregnant with twins, and then loses one twin in the early stages of pregnancy. While doctors and loved ones might encourage her to think of how lucky she is to have the ongoing pregnancy, she might be very sad about the loss of the other twin. Many fertility patients worry that they will not be able to get pregnant again, and minimizing the loss of this second child can make them feel even more alone in their grief.

Your ILO may go through all the stages of grief at various points in her fertility treatments. She may be sad and angry and depressed. She may be surprised or disconsolate. She may want to get together over a bottle of wine to discuss it with you, or she may want to hide under the covers and not speak to anyone. As usual, offer your support, but do not press her for any particular kind of reaction. Be a careful listener. If your ILO feels like she needs to grieve, grieve with her. Take her loss as seriously as you would the death of any close relative. Just because your ILO did not give birth to a child does not mean the child did not fully exist in her mind.

Takeaway Tip: *Respect your ILO's grief at all points in her journey toward parenthood.*

CHAPTER 19

Understand Third-Party Reproduction

If your ILO confides that she is considering egg donation, sperm donation, or a gestational carrier, you can best support her by understanding a little about what these terms mean and what the differences between them are. These third parties to reproduction fall into two categories—women who carry the child, and women and men who donate genetic material to make a child your ILO (or another woman) will carry.

In the first category are gestational carriers and traditional surrogates. A surrogate is a woman who volunteers and/or is compensated to be inseminated with the sperm of the male partner. Her own eggs are fertilized, but the child is always intended to be the child of the couple that engages her for her services. Given the ethical and legal issues involved, traditional surrogacy is largely a historical footnote, and has mostly been replaced by egg donation in combination with a gestational carrier.

A gestational carrier is a woman who carries an embryo that a couple has created through IVF, usually using the genetic material of each partner. The gestational carrier is not genetically related to the child.

The second category includes men and women who donate genetic material—either sperm or eggs. What leads hopeful parents to use an egg donor or sperm donor? Remember all that testing the male and female partners had to go through when they visited the reproductive endocrinologist? Well, sometimes that specialist can tell right away that there is a serious problem with one or both partners. Sometimes the male partner's sperm count is so low that pregnancy is almost impossible, even with

IVF and special micromanipulation techniques. Sometimes genetic testing will show that both partners are carriers for terrible genetic diseases. Sometimes it takes several failed IVF cycles to determine that the eggs or sperm are highly unlikely to work in the creation of a baby. In these cases, your ILO may choose a sperm or egg donor, and may sometime need to combine the donation with a gestational carrier to finally have a child with a genetic link to at least one intended parent.

Your ILO will certainly consider adoption at this point, and will also consider living child-free. But sometimes, after she and/or her partner have grieved the loss of their genetics, they decide that they want the experience of pregnancy, or they want to preserve one partner's genetics, or they investigate adoption and realize they are not good candidates or cannot risk the logistical and emotional vagaries of that process.

All these new ways to be a parent can feel overwhelming to you, and the way you talk about them can really make a difference to your ILO. Never refer to a traditional surrogate or a gestational carrier as the child's mother. Never refer to the sperm donor or egg donor as the parent. If third-party reproduction feels like a brave new world to you, educate yourself more, and ask questions without judgment. And if your ILO or her surrogate or gestational carrier does get pregnant, celebrate that pregnancy just as much as any other.

· ·

Takeaway Tip: Strive to understand surrogacy, egg donation, sperm donation, and gestational carriers if your ILO is considering them.

· ·

CHAPTER 20

Remember Your Infertile Loved One's Struggle with Infertility through Pregnancy and Beyond

When your ILO gets pregnant, you may think the special challenges of supporting her through infertility no longer apply. After all, wasn't pregnancy what all this was about? Well, many women experience fear and anxiety during pregnancy, and women who used to be infertile are no exception. In fact, your ILO may feel more anxiety about pregnancy, both about miscarrying and about the health of her child, than a woman who has conceived without difficulty. She may even feel guilty about complaining about pregnancy symptoms or the emotional and social changes that will come with motherhood.

While I did not feel restricted about complaining about my constant nausea, I myself had so much anxiety about my ultimately productive pregnancy that I wouldn't let anyone throw me a baby shower until my third trimester.

You can help your ILO by giving her space to share concerns with you. If she says something like, "I know I shouldn't complain about nausea, since pregnancy is exactly what I wanted," you can help her by saying, "You have just as much right to complain about pregnancy symptoms as anyone else!" Then go get her a ginger ale and some crackers.

This same advice applies once your ILO has given birth to a child. Women who have gone through IVF are actually more likely than other women to suffer from post-partum anxiety and depression. At the same time, they may be less likely to seek help, because they feel so grateful to have a baby at all. If your ILO does mention that she doesn't feel like she has a right to talk about negative emotions or sleep deprivation, you can help her by reminding her that her journey to parenthood was longer than many others, and that she deserves just as much support as any other new parent, if not more. You can remind her that the early months of motherhood are difficult even for a woman who got pregnant after a night of tequila shots and the music of Barry White, and that a woman who has gone through fertility treatments has possibly spent years of her life being tired and hormonal before she confronts this latest challenge.

You can help. Prepare a home-cooked meal or deliver some delicious take-out. Offer to hold the baby or do some dishes while your ILO gets some sleep.

••

Takeaway Tip: Remember your ILO's struggle with infertility affects her throughout pregnancy and even after.

••

CHAPTER 21

Respect Your Infertile Loved One's Decision to Stop Pursuing Parenthood

Some fertility patients will decide at some point that they no longer wish to try to have children. Some will attempt IVF, and third-party reproduction, and the adoption process without success, and will then decide that putting the majority of their energy into trying to become a parent is bad for their relationships and their personal mental (and perhaps physical) health. Others will decide to stop trying to be parents without pursuing any of these options. If you have spent a great deal of time supporting your ILO's decision to pursue fertility treatments, third-party reproduction, and/or adoption, it can be a big shift to support her decision to live without children.

You know all that your ILO has gone through in trying to become a parent, so you know that she did not make this decision without a lot of thought. You do not need to list all the reasons children are a burden or all the freedoms she has gained in making this decision. In fact, listing such reasons or denigrating parenthood may make her uncomfortable. Instead, you can simply reflect on all the emotional energy your ILO put into trying to be a parent, and hope that she finds peace in her decision. And one of the best ways to help her is semantic. Rather than referring to her state as childless, refer to her as being *child-free*.

Takeaway Tip: Not all ILOs will end up with a child. If your ILO decides to stop treatment or stop the adoption process, respect your ILO's decision to live child-free.

CHAPTER 22

Celebrate Your Infertile Loved One as Mother, No Matter Her Path to Motherhood

Although some ILOs will decide to live child-free, many others will become mothers, even though they may not arrive at motherhood by the path they originally envisioned. No matter the genetic or gestational origin of her baby, celebrate your ILO as a mother. Some women feel complicated emotions about adoption or surrogacy or the participation of a gestational carrier. These women might mention that they don't "deserve" a baby shower, or that they don't want to register for baby gifts. You can help your ILO by gently encouraging her to let other people celebrate her new life as a mother, no matter her path to motherhood. You can also shield your ILO from any well-meaning person who might be tempted to refer to a birth mother or egg donor or surrogate as "the mother."

It's worth noting that these questions of third-party reproduction and adoption will follow your ILO around even if she was able to get pregnant using her own genetics. For example, if your ILO was able to get pregnant using her own genetics, you might be tempted to say something like, "I'm so glad you got to have your own baby." You might be genuinely overjoyed to see your ILO's smile reflected in this new person. You might be thrilled to see pieces of both your ILO and her partner melded in a perfect new package. Your ILO might agree with you right away, but she might also have a bit of a mixed reaction to statements like these. She may agree with you, and feel happy that you supported her in her decision to pursue fertility treatments. But she may also feel like having a child through adoption or egg donation would have been equally wonderful, and she may hesitate to say that this way was superior to one of those paths.

••

Takeaway Tip: *Celebrate your ILO's transition to motherhood, even if she is reluctant.*

••

AFTERWORD

Between 2007 and 2011, I went through a dozen IUIs, three rounds of IVF, three miscarriages, and extensive genetic and metabolic testing. I met with two adoption agencies, two adoption lawyers, and one adoption consultant. In 2010, I conceived twins with the help of IVF, and lost one around eleven weeks. In 2011, I gave birth to a boy, who today is a charming, energetic, and very verbal toddler. I very much wanted another child, so in 2013, I went through additional testing and another frozen embryo transfer, which failed. My husband and I were in the process of setting our calendar for our next frozen embryo transfer when I spontaneously and accidentally became pregnant with twins. As my friend Ida says, "Life is long and strange."

Still, this spontaneous pregnancy, which some might say proved that I wasn't as infertile as my doctors and I assumed, has never made me empathize any less with the struggles of infertile women. I will never forget the sadness of not being able to conceive a child, or the roller coaster of hope and disappointment that infertility treatment, miscarriage, and attempts at adoption brings. And I will also never forget the support I received from my family and friends during this time. I really learned everything about how to support an infertile loved one from the ways I was supported during this time.

ABOUT THE AUTHOR

Zahie El Kouri writes about infertility and immigrant culture, sharing her experience of surviving infertility through personal essays and articles that address with humor, intellect, and empathy the needs and concerns of infertile women.

Zahie has taught creative writing at the University of North Florida and the University of Oregon Law School, and legal writing at Santa Clara University and Florida Coastal School of Law. She holds a JD from Cornell Law School and an MFA in creative writing from New School University. Her work has appeared in *Ars Medica: A Journal of Medicine, the Arts, and Humanities, Mizna, Memoir Journal, Dinarzad's Children: An Anthology of Contemporary Arab American Fiction, Brain, Child: The Magazine for Thinking Mothers*, and FullGrownPeople.com. If you'd like to learn more about her experience as an infertility patient, as a parent, and as a writer, please visit www.zahieelkouri.com, and sign up for occasional updates.